C000193067

50 TIPS
TO HELP YOU
SLEEP WELL

50 TIPS TO HELP YOU SLEEP WELL

Summersdale Publishers Ltd
46 West Street
Chichester
West Sussex
PO19 1RP
UK

www.summersdale.com

Printed and bound in China

ISBN: 978-1-84953-401-7

Substantial discounts on bulk quantities of Summersdale books are available to corporations, professional associations and other organisations. For details contact Nicky Douglas by telephone: +44 (0) 1243 756902, fax: +44 (0) 1243 786300, or email: nicky@summersdale.com.

50 TIPS
TO HELP YOU
SLEEP WELL

Anna Barnes

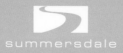

Introduction

Around 45 per cent of us will suffer with insomnia at some point in our lives. These fifty tips are designed to help you tackle sleep difficulties through simple, easy-to-implement techniques and lifestyle changes, and get you back to sleeping through the night. If you feel that insomnia is causing you too much difficulty, however, it is advised that you seek advice from your doctor.

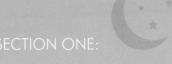

SECTION ONE:

STRESS AND SLEEP

When we are stressed, we do not sleep well, so eliminating or easing the causes of stress will have a direct positive impact on the quality of your sleep.

1

Identify and control the things that make you stressed

Over the course of two weeks, write down all the things that make you feel stressed, be they places, people or situations. Rate these stresses on a scale from one to ten, with one being only slightly stressful, and ten being the most stressful. Once you have identified your high-stress triggers you can take steps to eliminate them; for example, if getting the bus to work is a high-stress situation for you, try cycling or walking (which gives you the added benefit of extra exercise).

Practise mindfulness

Mindfulness is a technique for living in the here and now, rather than being preoccupied with the past or the future, which has developed from Buddhist teachings and can help your mind to prepare for a good night's sleep. Being mindful means living in the moment, and experiencing what is happening now. A simple way to start would be by altering your route to work slightly so that you pay more attention to your surroundings, rather than being 'on autopilot'. Taking time to reflect on your environment and situations can put your worries into perspective, where otherwise they might have preoccupied you and caused you stress.

3

Make a to-do list

Whether at work or at home, if you have lists of tasks going round in your head, this can cause stress and worry. The simple act of writing a to-do list and crossing each item off as it is done is very cathartic, and adds structure to your day-to-day life, helping you to feel organised and calm and giving your brain license to switch off when it comes to bedtime. Remember, you don't have to cross off every item; just making the list is progress in and of itself.

4

Write down your worries

We all have periods of worry – family, finance, career and health can all be sources of anxiety. Not being able to 'switch off' at night, and continuing to worry about different things, can cause sleep difficulties. Many people have lain awake at night at some point in their lives, thinking about that project that needs finishing, or the cat being at the vets. Writing these worries down allows you to voice them, helping you to think more clearly, and allowing you to sleep more easily. Some people find a further step helpful – to destroy the paper the worries are listed on by, for example, either ripping it up or throwing it into the fire – and seeing their worries move from their head, to the paper, and then away.

5

Talk to a friend or family member

If you think stresses and worries are making you sleep badly, or if you are just worried about how you have been sleeping, talking to someone close can be a huge help. Vocalising your concerns and hearing the reassurance and advice of someone whose opinions you trust can help alleviate anxiety and put you in a better position for restful sleep. If you do not have someone close to you to confide in, a counsellor or a service such as the Samaritans can provide the patient ear you seek.

6

Invest in some 'me time'

We often lead very busy lives, at work and at home. Taking a break to concentrate on yourself and how you are feeling is very beneficial in reducing stress levels and therefore helps to alleviate night-time worries. At work, breaking up your lunch hour across the day – two fifteen-minute breaks and one half-hour break – might work better for you. Using the smaller breaks to read the paper or just chat to colleagues will help you feel grounded. At home, taking the time in between tasks to sit down and call a friend, or read a chapter of a book, can help us not only to stay focussed, but to feel more positive too.

7

Enjoy the great outdoors

Being in natural surroundings can bring a real sense of tranquillity. Going for a walk by the sea or in the woods, or even just pottering in the garden, can improve your mood, ease muscle tension and lower blood pressure. When you feel close to nature it can give you the boost you need for restful sleep.

8

Exercise more

Going for a run, swim or bike ride isn't just good for your waistline – it's also great for getting healthy, restful sleep. As well as making your muscles tired, exercise helps your body use up stress hormones, like cortisol, which can make sleep difficult. Exercising in the afternoon or early evening will raise your body temperature and metabolism; when your core temperature drops again after around five hours you will feel naturally drowsy and find it easier to fall asleep.

9

Laugh more

The old adage tells us that 'laughter is the best medicine'. In many ways, this is true. Laughter helps us feel relaxed – it relieves tension and makes us feel happier by triggering the release of naturally occurring endorphins. As a result, laughter strengthens your immune system, boosts your energy, reduces pain and protects you from the damaging effects of stress – all of which promote a good night's sleep. Try watching your favourite comedy, swapping funny stories with friends or looking at a funny website for a bit of light relief.

10

Choose your times wisely

It can be tempting, when we are winding down after a busy day, to want to discuss everything with our partner in bed, or perhaps with friends via an online chat or the phone. Discussing your worries is a great idea, but it is best done earlier in the evening. Choosing to start a serious conversation about a topic of concern, such as health or finance, shortly before your planned time to go to sleep, will keep the subject fresh in your mind and may interfere with your ability to fall asleep and enjoy restful sleep. Instead, make a mental note to talk about it the next day, when you are feeling awake and refreshed.

SECTION TWO:

THE PSYCHOLOGY OF SLEEP

Sometimes it can be our own expectations and errant thoughts which make it hard for us to sleep soundly. Simple techniques such as positive thought can help combat this.

11

Make your
expectations realistic

Many of us lie awake at night worrying that we won't get the recommended eight hours of sleep that we need to function well. However, the 'worry' part of this scenario is what has the biggest negative effect. Studies have shown that most people will have no problem functioning with six or seven hours' sleep, and further, that if you have lost sleep, you only need to catch up about a third of the lost time to get back to normal; so, for example, if you went to bed an hour and a half late one night of the week, a thirty-minute lie-in at the weekend would do the trick.

Changing our perceptions of the time we need to sleep can help us feel more secure, and therefore help us sleep more easily, with a better quality of sleep.

Remember not to worry about the time

As well as setting ourselves unrealistic goals for how long we should sleep, many of us feel that we have been lying awake for far longer than we have. What may seem like hours as we are waiting for sleep to come is more likely to be just twenty to thirty minutes. In the same way, when we remember waking several times during the night, it is likely that we have lost no more than a few minutes' sleep at the most.

It is also worth remembering that simply lying down in a relaxed position is very beneficial in itself, and is a good step towards sleep.

Although it may take you some time to fall asleep, acknowledging that it is not going to take hours can ease the pressure many feel of not being able to drift off immediately. Feeling freer and less pressured can improve both the quantity and quality of sleep.

13

Use affirmations

An affirmation is a positive phrase you use to help change negative beliefs to positive ones. Affirmations work well when written down, and when said out loud. A positive affirmation to help you change your sleeping habits could be, 'I sleep well every night' or 'I fall asleep with ease'. It is important that the affirmation focusses on the positive outcome you want, rather than the negative you do not want. You can buy CDs of positive affirmations to listen to before sleep, or download them from the Internet, should you prefer.

14

The the the the the

Sometimes the mind refuses to be quiet. In these cases, repeating a word which doesn't mean anything can help clear your mind of thoughts and, helpfully, induce boredom. One recommendation is to use the word 'the', as this is short and means nothing on its own, though you can choose any word you think will work for you. Try repeating the word in your head every two seconds for five to ten minutes and let your mind be soothed into sleep.

15

Count sheep!

The idea of visualisation may sound 'New Age' to some, but people have been using it for many years. The old advice of 'count sheep until you fall asleep' is a form of visualisation – you see the sheep jumping over the fence one by one and count them, feeling sleepier as the numbers get higher.

Other visualisations may help. One suggestion would be, rather than visualising energetic sheep bouncing over a fence, why not visualise sleeping sheep? See yourself floating over a night-time meadow, passing dozing sheep one at a time. The more sheep you see, the more you want to lie down in the soft grass and rest. These sleeping sheep may help you get to sleep better than their wide-awake counterparts.

16

Let your worries float away

This is another form of visualisation which will help when seemingly insurmountable worries start circling round in your mind at night. If your mind is racing, looking for a solution it can't find, tell yourself, 'I can't do anything practical to help this today – I can think about it in the morning.' As you give your mind this message, see your worry trapped inside a colourful balloon, floating up and away, out of reach and out of mind.

17

Don't try to sleep

Research has shown that for many people with sleeping difficulties, the biggest problem is trying to go to sleep. When we put the emphasis on trying, and focus hard on falling asleep, treating it like a task, we actually make ourselves more awake. The act of focussing on and bringing attention to our inability to sleep is also likely to promote worry and exacerbate the problem. Instead, try not thinking about falling asleep, but rather decide that you only want to rest. Allow yourself to relax and enjoy being restful. Chances are you will fall asleep before you know it!

THE BEST ENVIRONMENT FOR HEALTHY SLEEP

If you find it hard to sleep, your bedroom can become an uninviting place. Making your bedroom a healthy and enticing environment is a great way to improve sleeping patterns.

Choose bed linen that makes you feel good

This doesn't just mean linen that looks pretty, though of course, having bed linen that reflects your personal taste will make you feel at home and comfortable. There is, however, slightly more to it than that.

Choosing the right bed linen for you means choosing something that will make you feel cosy and ready to sleep in the evening, and fresh and ready to go in the morning. For some people, cool cotton sheets and duvet covers work best. Others find silk gentler against their skin. For many people, synthetics cause them to sweat too much in the night, which can cause night-time waking. Invest in a couple of sets of good linen, rather than multiple cheap and cheerful sets of polyester sheets, and see how much more easily you fall asleep.

19

Cleanliness and sleepiness

Once you have found your ideal linen, it is important to keep it clean. Many people do not change their bed linen often enough, yet sleeping in fresh linen could help improve any sleep difficulties.

Bed linen should be washed at least once per week and thoroughly dried before being used again. Having two sets of linens makes this easier, as you can have one on the bed whilst the other is washed, dried, and stored, then swap at the end of the week. If you have the option of line-drying your linens in the fresh air, they become one of life's little luxuries – the scent of freshly wind-blown sheets is a real tonic. Routine can help you to keep your bed linen in top condition for optimal sleeping. For example, it could be part of your Sunday morning routine to strip off your bed linens ready for laundering and put the new sheets on.

Remember, if you have had a bout of illness, or a particularly hot night, change and wash the sheets more frequently to maintain a fresh and relaxing bed environment.

Look after your mattress

A mattress, like anything we use regularly, will eventually wear out and need replacing. Guidelines vary on how often you should get a new mattress, with some saying as little as five years, and others as long as ten. Essentially, each person is unique and will need to replace their mattress at different times. Factors such as weight loss or gain, pregnancy, and frequency of use will inform how often you need to change yours.

To help keep your mattress in good shape, it is wise to turn it over or rotate it every few months. Of course, if you can feel any loose springs through the mattress when you lay on it, or if it sags in the place you generally sleep, it is time for a replacement. Careful consideration should be given to mattress choice as, though a good mattress will often have a higher price, it is likely to last longer, and the long-term benefit of good sleep is worth it. Get a new mattress that's right for you and you may have the best sleep you've had in quite some time.

21

Consider changing your pillow

Many of us sleep on pillows that are too old, too hard or too soft. Getting a new pillow, or changing the type of pillow that you use, can help you get to sleep more easily at bedtime, as well as improving the quality of your sleep. By investing in a pillow designed for your sleep-type, you can save money in the long run as you will only need one pillow rather than the two or three that most of us use, and it will most likely be made from longer-lasting material.

While most of us will use either down- or hollow-fibre-filled pillows, memory-foam pillows with special dips and raised edges can be found in many specialist bed shops and home retailers — some are designed for those who sleep on their back, others for those who sleep on their sides. It may seem odd at first after being used to soft, pliant pillows, but the more supportive variety will hold your head and neck in the right way, allowing for a more comfortable position, and sounder sleep.

Find ways to make your night quieter

Night-time noise can be a big cause of sleep disturbance. This can be anything from a ticking clock, to sirens, to a snoring partner. It is likely you will already know which noises are the most likely to wake you up. In an ideal world, you would remove these sounds completely, but of course, this is not always possible. Things you can do, however, like removing the battery from a ticking clock at night or fixing that dripping tap, will do much to help the quality of your sleep improve.

23

Make your bedroom
your sanctuary

Experts say that our bed should be for sleeping and sex only. Keeping the bed as a work- and life-stress-free zone will help your body and mind to identify it as a place of rest, relaxation, enjoyment and, ultimately, sleep. To do this, it is a good idea to free your room of computers and televisions – anything that will make you tempted to watch some late-night videos! – and make your bedroom tidy and inviting; a safe, cocoon-like environment. Do any paperwork in another room and keep important discussions out of the bedroom. You'll soon be sleeping more soundly!

24

Ways to combat noise

Two of the main methods for dealing with excess noise are very simple, and have been shown to be very effective. The first, earplugs, have been used for many years for everything from working in loud factories to shutting out the world on long plane journeys. Earplugs can be purchased cheaply, and block out those unwanted noises. The second, white noise machines, can be pricy. You can, however, buy CDs of white noise to play to yourself, or get white noise generator apps for your smartphone or tablet. Many people find this kind of noise soothing, blocking out all other noises and helping them to fall asleep more easily, and to sleep more soundly.

25

Keep it dark

Light is a big cause of disturbed sleep and early waking. While darkness causes your brain to produce melatonin, a hormone that makes you feel sleepy, light helps it produce serotonin, too much of which will make you feel more awake.

To help keep your bedroom as dark as possible, make sure any electrical items such as stereos are turned off, not on standby, as the lights from their displays may keep you awake. You should also choose thick, dark curtains or blinds, to ensure outside light does not intrude and wake you. If light is a particular nuisance for you, try using blackout curtains or blinds in your bedroom.

Keep your room cool

Although many describe sleep as warm and comfortable, being too warm will make it difficult for you to stay asleep. Avoid leaving the heating on in your bedroom, even on very chilly evenings, as this will make the air too warm and you may become sweaty in the night. If possible, leave a window slightly open to allow the cool night air to moderate your room temperature. If the noise of nearby traffic is too disturbing for you, perhaps a quiet fan or more lightweight bedding will do the trick. Your bedroom should only be around 16°C, and well ventilated, helping you sleep restfully through the night.

RELAXATION TECHNIQUES AND SELF-HYPNOSIS

One of the key ways to ensure a good night's sleep is by being relaxed. Simple relaxation techniques can be practised every day and make a very positive difference to sleep, and to general wellbeing.

Relax – breathe

Many of us use a good portion of the time we could be using for relaxing in the pursuit of non-sleep-inducing activities such as completing extra work, discussing issues with our partner or family, or simply worrying about what has happened today, and what is going to happen tomorrow. We simply do not, or cannot, switch off. This widespread problem is one you will need to combat to help you sleep soundly.

Learning to relax is both simple and complex at the same time. Whilst we know we just have to stop, our minds race away, and we are left chasing them. A simple way to start training your body to relax in the evenings is to practise mindful deep breathing. Close your eyes and focus on your breath. Think only about your breath, and the way it feels coming into your body and then out. Once you are fully aware of your breathing, try taking deeper breaths, breathing in for a count of six and out for a count of six. Stay focussed on your breath. Do this for five minutes shortly before bed and you should feel more relaxed, and ready for sleep.

Give yoga a try

Yoga is an ancient form of exercise which originated in India. It has become very popular in the last few years, and with good reason. Not only is yoga a gentle form of exercise, which in and of itself can help the body to release stress and be more ready for sleep, but it also promotes relaxation. Yoga practice combines movements with breathing, so that the mind is focussed on what the body is doing. This physical focus helps the mind to relax, to stop thinking about the worries of the day. A good class will also end with yogic sleep, or progressive relaxation, helping both mind and body slow down and truly relax.

Progressive relaxation

Not just for the yoga class, progressive relaxation is a great tool for everyday use. The theory is that if you focus intensely on each part of the body, and then let it go, you will relax more completely than if you were to simply 'try' to relax. There are many different forms of progressive relaxation, some using affirmations or mantras, and some focussing on the physical body.

One of the simplest methods you can use, and an easy way to introduce yourself to progressive relaxation, is to lie in bed, on your back, ready to go to sleep. Starting with your toes, and working your way slowly up your body to your head, tightly clench your muscles and hold them for five seconds, then release. The effect will be greater if you clench on your in-breath, and release on your out-breath. If you find your mind wandering, try using the mantra, 'I am relaxing my toes, I can feel my toes completely relaxed', repeating for each body part. You can even find apps to help you through the process. By the end, you should feel physically and mentally relaxed, and ready for sleep.

30

Meditate on it

Meditation has been used by many cultures around the world for centuries. Yoga is described as a 'moving meditation', showing that this practice takes many forms. You don't necessarily have to sit cross-legged and chant mantras to meditate, though you can if you find it helpful.

Put simply, meditation is a way of quieting your mind, and allowing yourself time to be still. A good way to start, if meditation is new to you, is to sit in a comfortable position with a straight back, resting your palms face-up in your lap. Close your eyes and focus on one of your senses. When your mind begins to wander, gently bring it back to your chosen sense. Doing this for five to ten minutes before you settle down to sleep can leave you feeling relaxed and refreshed, and lead to easier sleep.

Guided meditation

As its name suggests, this is a form of meditation in which, rather than you taking the lead, someone else is guiding you. If you find sitting still with your own thoughts difficult, this could be for you. It is also more structured than self-led meditation, which can make it easier to follow.

Guided meditation may be done in a class setting; look in to your local natural health centres or yoga studios to see if they run classes. Alternatively, you can buy CDs of guided meditation, or download meditation tracks from the Internet. However you choose to do it, this is a great way to feel relaxed quickly, and has long-lasting after-effects, helping you feel relaxed into the next day.

SECTION FIVE:
HEALTHY HABITS

Getting into bad habits often seems much easier than adopting good ones. Try using these habit-forming techniques to build up healthy sleeping practice.

Sleep schedule

One of the things which can be most damaging to our sleeping patterns is a lack of routine. Many of us will go to bed at midnight on a weekday, trying to finish off some task or other, and then wake at six. Then, at the weekend, we will likely go to bed later but sleep in until late in the morning in a bid to 'catch up' with sleep. The best thing is to not feel the need for this catching up in the first place. To combat this, try to go to bed and wake at around the same time each day. If you aim to not vary by more than an hour each way, this will help to keep your body clock working at its optimum level.

When your body clock associates certain times of the day with waking or sleeping, it produces the relevant hormone: serotonin to help keep you awake, or melatonin to help you sleep. Drastically changing your bedtime and the length of time you sleep day-to-day confuses the body and makes hormone production irregular, which in turn makes it harder to get a good night's sleep. So keep your hours regular, and you will keep your hormone production regular too.

33

Bedtime routines

There are many ways to get ready for bed, and for each person, different activities make them feel more awake, or sleepier. Many people find taking a warm bath, scented with relaxing oils or bath products such as lavender or sandalwood, very relaxing at night. For some, reading a good book last thing at night will send them off; for others, a warm drink before bed is the thing. What they have in common though is that they are part of a routine, and act as triggers, telling our body and mind that it is now time to sleep.

If you have never had a routine, try out some of the tips in this book. Some will work better for you than others – try to incorporate these every day. As you build your routine, your body will come to expect these pre-sleep actions, and will automatically start getting sleepier as you start your routine.

34

Don't spend too long in bed

Restricting the time you spend in bed may seem like the opposite of what you want to do if you are having trouble sleeping. It is easy to think that the longer you stay in bed, the more likely it is you will get some sleep. However, this is often not the case. Being in bed and unable to get to sleep or stay asleep can cause frustration or worry, which in turn will make sleep quality worse, causing a vicious cycle.

At first, try to work out how many hours you actually sleep out of those you spend in bed, and try only going to bed for that length of time. If, for example, you sleep for five hours a night and have to be up at seven, you should go to bed at two in the morning. This may sound very late, but by only being in bed for your sleeping hours, you will be teaching your body that bed is for sleep. When you are sleeping for 90 per cent of the time you spend in bed, you can start to increase the hours you spend there, until you are sleeping comfortably through the night.

Increase the time you spend in bed, slowly but surely

Once you have put the previous tip into action, you will most likely want to start increasing the hours you spend in bed, so as to increase the hours you spend asleep. This should be done gradually, as you want to ensure your body and mind still associate the bed with sleep. Try adding half an hour at a time to your bedtime. Once you are sure you are sleeping for 90 per cent of the time you are in bed again, you can add another half an hour, and so on, until you have reached the point when you are sleeping the amount that is ideal for you to feel rested. Remember, this will vary from person to person, and you are the best judge of how much is right for you.

36

Are you feeling sleepy?

Although it is good to identify your ideal bedtime, based on the number of hours you sleep, it is equally important to only go to bed once you are feeling sleepy. Many of us are tired once we finish work, study or an exercise regime, but this does not equate to being sleepy. Signs of being sleepy include heavy eyelids, yawning and difficulty concentrating – our bodies telling us that we are ready for sleep. If you are not feeling sleepy at your bedtime, your bedtime routine should help. Going to bed before you are sleepy can lead to difficulty falling asleep, and early waking, so it is best avoided.

37

If you can't sleep, get out of bed

We know that we want to associate bed with sleep, so, when unable to sleep, it is often a good idea to get up and move out of the bedroom. Try doing an activity which will soothe you, such as reading a book in soft light, or listening to gentle music, as this will help you to feel sleepy again. However, you should avoid switching on bright overhead lights or watching TV, as this will stimulate your brain and signal that it is time to be awake.

FOOD AND SLEEP

The way we eat and drink affects our body in many ways. Some foods are said to be good for the heart, or the brain, while others aid digestion. But the way you eat and drink could also be having a direct effect on the way you sleep.

A balanced diet

Before turning to the specific foods which aid sleep, it is important to ensure you are having a balanced diet from which to start. Eating the right amount of calories for your age, height and sex, and ensuring you get enough proteins, fibre and vitamin-rich vegetables, will give you a good basis for general health, and should improve digestion, which will aid sleep in and of itself.

Don't snack just before bed

Eating directly before you go to sleep can cause sleep disturbance as your body tries to digest your meal. Digestion, like all bodily functions, slows down during sleep, so the food will take longer than usual to pass through your digestive system, and may be stored as fat rather than used for energy. It is generally advised that you eat your last meal at least two hours before you go to bed, giving your body time to digest before you lie down for your night's rest.

If you have to snack, be a fan of tryptophan

Some of us have a snack before bed as part of our bedtime routine. If you are in this group of people and feel your snack is part of a routine that helps you get to sleep, then make sure you are snacking on the right things. Tryptophan is an amino acid which is used by the body in its production of serotonin. Serotonin is the 'happy' hormone which, in the right amounts, helps keep us calm and relaxed, and it in turn is part of the body's melatonin-production process. If you must eat before bedtime, keep to a small snack and, most importantly, try to snack on tryptophan-rich foods such as bananas, as these can actually aid sleep.

Low GI for better sleep

You may have heard about the health benefits a low-GI diet can have for you – more steady energy levels, less bloating, no sugar cravings – but eating a low-GI diet can also be beneficial for your sleep quality. GI stands for Glycaemic Index – the ranking of carbohydrate-containing foods based on their overall effect on blood glucose levels. When we eat foods with a high GI, such as white bread, pastries and sweets, our blood sugar spikes and then drops rapidly, leaving us tired, irritable and hungry. This can continue on into the night, so if you have finished the evening off with sweetened tea and biscuits, you can wake in the night with feelings of hunger. Eating low-GI foods helps ensure your body is fuelled throughout the night, meaning you don't get the midnight snack-attack and have steadier sleep.

42

Magnesium, 'nature's tranquiliser'

Magnesium is an essential nutrient which helps the body function well, particularly when it comes to sleep. A lack of this mineral has been linked to early waking. Magnesium helps you to relax, calming the mind and the body, and can alleviate night cramps. Recommended daily intakes of magnesium are 270 g for men and 300 g for women, all of which you can get from a balanced diet. Magnesium-rich foods include dark green leafy vegetables such as spinach or broccoli, nuts, beans, herbs and oats. Eat plenty and reap the benefits.

43

Calcium isn't just for teeth and bones

Like magnesium, good levels of calcium in the body are said to help promote restful sleep. Two thousand milligrams is enough calcium for an adult – try not to have too much more than this, as it can interfere with the uptake of other minerals, such as iron, and leave you feeling flat.

Calcium is found in dairy foods, though many people find these hard to digest, meaning uptake is not always optimal. Dairy foods do also contain tryptophan which can aid sleep, and a small drink of warm milk is often helpful when trying to sleep. Other calcium sources include green leafy vegetables such as purple sprouting broccoli or kale, brazil nuts, lentils, seeds, dried apricots and figs. Even tap water, especially in hard-water areas, contains calcium.

44

B vitamins for health and happiness

B vitamins are essential for maintaining a healthy nervous system, and for ensuring sound sleep. Most B vitamins are found in abundance in a balanced diet, but certain ones, such as B12, can be harder to obtain through your food. Eating fortified breakfast cereals can help you get your daily dose of B vitamins, as can yeast-based spreads such as Marmite. If you are concerned that you may not be getting enough of these essential vitamins, it may be worth investing in a daily B-vitamin complex to supplement your diet.

45

Drinking before bed

It is usually not a good idea to drink a large amount before going to sleep, as you may be woken up with a full bladder in the night. Even if it does not wake you completely, the likelihood is that the discomfort of a full bladder will stop you from sleeping restfully through the night. You shouldn't cut out water, however, as dehydration can also cause sleep problems. It may suit you to have a glass of water by your bed, for you to sip as and when needed.

Many people will have a 'nightcap' before bed, believing that a small alcoholic drink helps send them to sleep. This is true to a certain extent, as alcohol does have a sedative effect, but once this initial effect has worn off it acts as a stimulant and may disturb the later, deeper stages of sleep, leaving you feeling unrested in the morning. If you must have a nightcap, opt for a small glass of Chianti, Merlot or Cabernet Sauvignon, as the grape skins used in these wines are rich with the sleep hormone, melatonin. Do make sure it is a small one, though!

Anyone for tea?

Many people like to finish the day with a warm drink before bed, and this is an excellent idea. However, a habit of drinking caffeine-rich tea and coffee before going to sleep will undoubtedly have a negative effect on your sleep.

Caffeine is a strong stimulant found not only in coffee and tea but also in colas and energy drinks. Too much of any of these will negatively impact on the quality of your sleep. Instead, try a soothing caffeine-free herbal tea such as chamomile, lemon balm or valerian. You can even get specially blended bedtime teas to gently help you to sleep.

Caffeine switch

Caffeine and similar stimulants should also be avoided as much as possible during the day. It can be tempting if you are tired after a poor night's sleep to reach for a cup of caffeine-rich coffee or cola, but your body will thank you if, instead, you go for water or antioxidant-rich green tea. The caffeine you drink during the day has long-lasting after-effects and can interfere with your ability to get to sleep. Water, on the other hand, helps to flush toxins from your body, as does green tea. A healthy body free from toxins will feel less tired during the day, and sleep better at night.

SECTION SEVEN:

THE MEDICAL SIDE OF THINGS

If sleep difficulties are causing you problems that the previous tips are not tackling, a medical approach should be taken. Your GP can advise you on what is best for your case in particular.

48

Talk to your doctor about sleep disorders

You may find that the more holistic approaches don't completely resolve your sleep problems. In this case, you may be suffering from a sleep disorder which needs medical treatment before you will be able to sleep well. Disorders are usually categorised by which aspect of your sleep-related health they affect: breathing, movement, circadian rhythm, parasomnias (such as sleepwalking) or hypersomnias (such as narcolepsy).

Talking with your doctor about your symptoms will help them to give you a diagnosis and work out the best course of treatment for you. Sometimes sleeping tablets may be prescribed, but this is a short-term measure and should only be considered to get your sleep back into a normal rhythm so that other treatments can be more effective.

Consider complementary therapies

Many complementary therapies are now supported by doctors, though exactly what is available to you will depend on where you live. If you feel an alternative therapy such as acupuncture, aromatherapy or homeopathy may be of help and interest to you, speak to your doctor about your options.

If you live in an area where complementary therapies are not widely available on the NHS, check out your local natural health centres or even community centres. Many places will offer low-cost initial sessions so that you can see if a particular therapy is right for you before embarking on a course of treatments.

And finally...
keep a sleep diary

Keeping a simple sleep diary, recording when and how often you wake, and how long for, can help you find the root causes of your sleeping problems. Keep it simple (a notebook or just a plain piece of paper will do), and don't worry if you are only using approximate timings – the last thing you need is the stress of clock-watching when you are already having trouble sleeping. This diary will help you to identify and therefore work on the causes of your sleeplessness.

The Patient UK website has a downloadable sleep diary which you can print out and keep by your bed, as well as an iPhone app. Just go to their website (www.patient.co.uk) and type 'sleep diary' into the search box.

Notes

50 TIPS
TO HELP YOU
DE-STRESS

Anna Barnes

50 TIPS TO HELP YOU DE-STRESS

Anna Barnes

ISBN: 978-1-84953-402-4

Hardback

£5.99

No matter how hard we try, there are times for all of us when the stresses and strains of daily life start to pile up. This book of simple, easy-to-follow tips gives you the tools and techniques you need to recognise your stress triggers and learn to take life as it comes, with a calm and balanced outlook.

If you're interested in finding out more about our books,
find us on Facebook at **Summersdale Publishers**
and follow us on Twitter at **@Summersdale**.

www.summersdale.com